William Kergroach

Autism

William Kergroach

Autism

How to make an autistic boy happy

JustFiction Edition

Cover image: www.ingimage.com

Publisher:
JustFiction! Edition
is a trademark of
Dodo Books Indian Ocean Ltd. and OmniScriptum S.R.L publishing group

120 High Road, East Finchley, London, N2 9ED, United Kingdom
Str. Armeneasca 28/1, office 1, Chisinau MD-2012, Republic of Moldova, Europe
Printed at: see last page
ISBN: 978-3-659-47037-0

How to make an autistic boy happy

The simple and complete guide

William Kergroach

A few words from a Dad

A few years ago, I had already written a book on autism. I tried to summarize everything I had read and experienced on the subject. I was trying to save you time, to tell you everything we knew about autism.

And then the years passed. Stanislas has grown up, and so have we, his parents.

Today, I think that my son will probably not be completely cured. We met with specialists, endured a lot of fools, incompetents, pretentious people, egomaniacs and medical psychopaths who had power over poor, beleaguered parents and a kid in trouble.

We also met some good people. We were fortunate to come across dedicated doctors, competent and modest professionals.

In the end, in addition to the skills of the specialists, the discoveries of science, we realized that autism required skills that were broader than the solutions that the socio-medical world could provide.

My goal today, more than hoping for a miraculous cure for Stanislas, is that he be a happy boy. I therefore go back to my initial text,

I note what we have observed about all the much vaunted "methods".
My question remains: why inflict on our child, and on ourselves, drastic diets, severe diets, uncomfortable treatments, overloaded schedules, multiple prohibitions, in order to have, in the end, a child who will never be "normal"?
The arrival of a child with a disability in a family is a trial for everyone: for the child, for his brothers and sisters, his parents and the family.
It is also an opportunity to change perspective, to reflect on our life, on our certainties, on the meaning of our passage on earth. A disabled child is a chance for our soul as parents. Some people understand what I mean.
Our goal today is to never see the smile disappear from the face of our Stanislas, from the face of his brothers and sisters and from our faces as father and mother. Our goal is to remain a strong and loving couple that does not sink into exhaustion and despair. This is a reality we see all too often in the faces of many parents of children with disabilities.
So, far from the books of doctors and specialists, far from the (dismal) promises of all the "gurus" in the field, I hope to save you time, or not to waste any. The purpose of this book is to help

you reach the right mental and spiritual disposition to remain serene and to transmit this peace and satisfaction to your children.
In the end, it's about having happy and fulfilled children, and parents who grow up and appreciate the opportunity for mental and spiritual evolution that is offered to them. Because, yes, a child is an opportunity for evolution for the parents.
This is the teaching of this book, which teaches you how to make a (autistic) child happy by radiating love, relaxation and humor.
The book is especially intended for young parents, who are discovering their child's disability and will take years to understand and accept this ordeal. If my book allows you to come to the necessary conclusions more quickly and allows you to escape the medical delusion and the therapy fanatics as much as possible. I have written this book to help you understand that it is as much about protecting your child as it is about helping her progress. If you can get past some of the crazy people who want to take over your life, that will be a benefit.
That said, for the perfectionists, the dynamic ones, the fighters, I have reviewed all the methods, it is up to you.

I wish you a useful reading to live years of happiness with your family.

What is autism?

Autism is a behavioral disorder, you are told. The term is, however, applied to a multitude of behavioral "abnormalities. There are a thousand kinds of autism!

The disorder is not psychological in origin, not triggered by the parents' attitude, love history or genes. It is, perhaps, an initial "fragility" of the individual, which is triggered by exposure to different factors. It is strongly suspected, for example, that the heavy metals in the vaccines administered to children since the 1980s and 1990s have played an important role in the explosion of the phenomenon.

One is born autistic in the same way as one has light or dark eyes.

Autism affects the ability to communicate and interact with others. People with autism perceive the world around them in a different way and find their own alternative strategies to deal with their own skills. These strategies, being different from the path chosen by "normal" people, can cause mutual misunderstanding and embarrassment. Fortunately, because our era is more sensitive to "difference" and "tolerant"

behaviors, it is much easier to be autistic or to have autistic children today than in the past!
Autism is now the fastest growing behavioral disorder in the world. So, since the phenomenon is growing, you might as well live it well and make your autistic child, whose case is less and less exceptional, as happy and fulfilled as possible.
As a parent, I will try to share with you what has worked for our child, for our other children, and for our couple. Beware, we are not a model family, I am not a super-Dad, super intelligent, patient, understanding, who will show you how I succeeded in everything for my autistic child, my family, my love life!
Far from being a specialist's book, with incomprehensible jargon, I have tried to speak a language that you will understand and to use terms and concepts that I myself understand.
With no double talk, no easy answers, no boasting, here is my simple testimony and my experience as a parent of an eleven year old child. We know that we are facing other challenges (puberty, our own aging, etc.) but I think we are relatively ready.
My child is not cured, he is getting better in some ways, other problems are and will be arising... He

will probably be autistic for the rest of his life, and it's going pretty well for us, because we've decided that it's going to be that way. We have learned that a certain philosophical and metaphysical approach, and a lot of humor and derision, can help us survive many difficulties. It is this mindset, more than anything, that I want to help you acquire.

Again, we had our moments of doubt, panic, exhaustion and discouragement. We don't have it all figured out, we don't know the future, and we undoubtedly have some complicated moments ahead of us.

So, here, there is no miracle recipe, but some useful tips to make things go smoothly.

What causes autism?

The causes are officially unknown. Few grants are given to researchers to work on this sensitive subject, because the American pharmaceutical industry knows that it has something to do with it... But, once again, several studies allow us to suspect that the administration of certain vaccines to babies can trigger autistic disorders. Well, once you say that, there's still no way to reverse it. Big Pharma won't let go of its money and it won't cure our children. So we have to move on!

It is said that it is a bad transmission between the reception and processing of information in the brain that causes the behavioral abnormality.

In autistic people, the growth of the brain and the way neurons are organized and connected are abnormal. The causes of autism are therefore genetic, with probably an environmental "trigger" (vaccines, pollution).

What is the behavior, in general, of an autistic person?

The autistic person isolates himself. Their relationship with others is disrupted by their inability to express themselves, to express emotions, to understand social codes, and to communicate in general.
The autistic person seems to have a limited interest in his surroundings, but he is not indifferent to them. As a parent, one can even observe a great deal of sensitivity to others, and especially to the "energy" they give off.
Some autistic people have repetitive behaviours, rituals, which can disturb you, your family and your immediate environment. This certainly affects your life in society. If you are the type of person who wants to present a smooth profile and a perfect appearance, you are screwed. So take a breath, sit back, reflect on your life and grow. This is a great opportunity for you to not remain a jerk and die having learned something from your journey on earth.
Again, it is difficult to characterize autism. The manifestations of autism vary greatly from person to person. They even vary in the same

person over a lifetime. What is certain is that a child with autism is a disruption of our public image and a real challenge for our personal history, the management of our emotions, our resilience to hardship, etc.

What are the first signs of autism?

The child does not babble at one year.
Does not talk at 18 months.
Does not associate words at 24 months.
Thereafter, his language is not developed, not sophisticated. Uses a singular tone of voice, with a characteristic intonation. Does not speak like other children.
He has a stare, which alerts your parenting instinct. Because, deep down, you realize it quickly.
The difficulty is to accept, to go beyond denial. We don't want our child to be less than his peers, it's normal. We feel a form of injustice. Why him, but especially why does this happen to me? Our entourage will either be extremely brutal or excessively reassuring. We all want to avoid seeing the obvious.
That's what you have to work on from the start.

At what age can autism be diagnosed?

A reliable diagnosis of autism can be made as early as 2 years of age. Then you see the medical community take hold of your baby. You will be sent from one department to another, from one specialist to another. These people recommend each other. You finance their lifestyle and their expenses of notables. Be careful not to say "amen" to everything. Your child's fate is your responsibility first. None of these specialists, who live on your drama, will cure your child.
At best, the most competent ones will help you to understand what is happening to you, to react correctly to your child's calls.
In any case, taking care of your child, and possible improvements, will take time. So don't rush and let every specialist see, and take money from you, to confirm what you already know.
Parents often spot "abnormalities" in their baby's behavior. But they are told that everything is fine, that it will change, that it depends on the children, etc.
Your intuition as a parent is always right. The diagnosis of the specialists is only a confirmation, in a very short time and with a

specialist's jargon, of what you observe on a daily basis.

How is autism diagnosed?

As there are many different types of autism, there is no single test that can be used to diagnose autism. Doctors use several tests that, when added together, help to establish performance.

The diagnosis of autism is based on a cluster of abnormalities observed in the child by parents and professionals.

A "mild" autistic person is one with autism disorders that are not too disabling: fairly good communication, neurological disorders that are not too severe, learning skills, etc. This type of autistic person is called a "high functioning" autistic person.

There are "heavy" autistic people, very handicapped in their daily life, their abilities, their behavior.

There are also Asperger's autistics. They are normally, even exceptionally, able, understand and express themselves correctly. Many of them, however, still have a little "quirky" side. Their love life remains complicated, due to their sensitivity or insensitivity to the emotions of

What are the communication problems of the autistic person?

The autistic person can speak, and even very well, but not always in an appropriate way. Either the tone is strange or the speech is inappropriate.
The autistic person has difficulty or is unable to ask for help, express his or her needs, the origin of his or her pain, etc.
One of the most common language disorders is echolalia: the systematic repetition of words or phrases. This is disconcerting for parents and family members. It is most often an expression of anxiety in the autistic person.
The autistic person also has problems understanding mimicry and gestures appropriate for life in society. This is why caregivers teach them to recognize the emotion of anger, contentment or fear in the faces of others.
It is difficult for the autistic person to imitate the gestures, expressions and codes of social life. It can even be said that they don't always seem to find it interesting...

How to behave with an autistic person?

As one should behave with everyone else: in a simple, spontaneous and balanced way. Autistic people, like many handicapped people, perceive very well our emotional imbalance, our aggressiveness, our hypocrisy, our superficiality. So, stay yourself, don't play a role, they will spot you very quickly...

Autistic people have difficulty expressing what they feel. Take the time to listen to them and help them express their feelings.

In case of a crisis, remain calm and reassuring. The autistic person is already having a hard time, so don't rush him/her. Try to help them by being calm and forgiving.

As with all children, bend down to their level. Speak slowly and, above all, gently.

Give simple instructions and repeat your request calmly. The autistic child may appear to be inattentive, with a peripheral gaze, for example, when he is interested. They are simply having difficulty. Be patient, empathetic and understanding.

If you can, use light physical contact, such as a touch of the hand, to reassure the person with autism.

Finally, give the person with autism time to process the information you wish to convey. This may sometimes seem a little long, but you must remember that the autistic person does not speak your language: he or she must translate what you ask.

How do you get an autistic person to eat?

Eating can be a big problem for an autistic person. It is frustrating for parents in particular.
You have to use strategies. You can try to insist that the autistic person eat something new or feared. They may end up being pleasantly surprised and embrace the novelty.
But this is tricky. It is important to avoid being stubborn and trying to force the autistic child, at the risk of triggering an anxiety attack and other problems later on.
Always offer him a food he likes with another he likes less or is not familiar with, and always in small quantities.
If you always serve the same food he likes, he may not want to eat it afterwards.
Diversify, as much as possible, the form of the food (purée, pieces, gratin...).
We have a sickly child at home. He loses weight for no reason, takes three hours to finish his meal...
We have adapted our method: we offer him food non-stop, all day long when he is at home.

What medication for autism?

No medication can cure autism. Some molecules can help the child sleep, make him/her calmer, improve his/her concentration, etc.

Be careful, get several opinions. In the end, it is always you, the parents, who must decide.

You can try, observe, interrupt or stop a medication. It is up to you to draw conclusions.

Beware of doctors, psychiatrists and other gurus who want to impose on you

Their character,

Their solutions,

Their certainties

And their miracle cures.

If they seem to lose interest in your child's case because you express doubts about their method, get rid of them.

There are too many unassailable "mandarins" and "spoiled children" in the medical profession! These people have the upper hand over us because they are connected to death and disease that terrorize us. These monsters of pride and fatuity know, more often than not, little of value. They speak with authority to reassure themselves of the legitimacy of their degree.

It is normal that we seek help when we are in difficulty, especially when our children are in danger. But the ordeal is yours, it will last your whole life. So you will have to rely on yourself.
Throughout your life as a parent of a child with a disability, if you haven't withdrawn into your own bubble like many stricken parents, you will meet many people. Some will help you, some will support you, some will give you a nightmare.
The more serene you are and the more you are committed to respecting yourself and your child, the less you will suffer from all the parasites generated by the medical and para-medical environment.

What percentage of the population is affected by autism?

Americans have been the first victims of the pharmaceutical industry, especially vaccines of course. American studies show that today one child out of 88 is affected by autism.
In Europe, we are already talking about one child in 100-150.
Men are over-represented: there are about 4 to 5 autistic boys for 1 girl.
The evolution of autism is exponential. More and more cases are being diagnosed. There is about a 10% increase in autism diagnoses each year.
This poses a major question to society. Obviously, there are going to be more and more autistic people among us. This should, in time, have consequences for the way we live together.
Unfortunately, too few politicians seem to be affected (too old to procreate perhaps) by this phenomenon. Handicap, and autism in particular, are not seriously addressed by politicians who do not see further than their term of office.
Too few structures are adapted, too few people are properly trained. The path of parents of

Techniques for learning?

An autistic person can be disturbed by :
A poster,
Sound stimuli,
Lights.
Headphones or earplugs can be used to reduce noise, if the autistic person is hypersensitive to noise.
A good position with armrests and footrests helps to capture the attention of the autistic person.
An object of the autistic person's choice, which he or she can handle or simply hold, should be tolerated at first during learning.
Remove all unnecessary objects from around an autistic person whose attention you want to capture.
Begin and end each work sequence with an activity that the autistic person has mastered and enjoys.
Similarly, alternate difficult tasks with more controlled tasks that reassure the autistic person.
Use visual aids, pictures, pictograms, to support the attention and understanding of an autistic person.
But, please, do not try to turn him into a trained

monkey! Your child is autistic, he is a handicapped person who has limits, accept it. If a skill is too difficult to learn, let it go, don't push it, please!

Competition and the desire for perfection must be based on voluntariness. Your child probably didn't make that choice. So stop making it a personal challenge. If you're a champion, if you've racked up awards and accolades for excellence, that's your story, that's your ego problem. Grow up.

On the other hand, if you succeed in making your autistic child happy and serene, that will be your greatest victory.

The different "methods"...

Whatever the discipline and the interest of each discipline, it is the quality of the human being that comes first. I have outlined what you should expect from each discipline.

Speech-Language Pathology

The speech-language pathologist helps to improve the communication skills of the autistic person, allowing him or her to
to better express their needs or desires.
The speech therapist should work with teachers, support staff, and most importantly, families.

Occupational Therapy

Occupational therapy is rehabilitation treatment to help the autistic person learn everyday movements, such as dressing, using utensils, cutting with scissors or writing. Beyond that, the

occupational therapist helps the autistic person improve his or her social behavior and gain independence.
The idea, with or without occupational therapy, is to offer the autistic person the possibility of reaching his or her full potential, while respecting his or her integrity, rhythm and well-being.
Remember: don't look for performance, but for your child's happiness.

Physiotherapy

Physiotherapy is used to improve gross motor skills and participate in daily activities such as walking, sitting, coordination and balance. It is a session that should be enjoyable for the child.

ABA therapy and similar methods

ABA stands for Applied Behavior Analysis. ABA is a behavioral approach that works to encourage positive behaviors and discourage negative ones.
For one child, a minimum of two educators take turns in a 2-3 hour session. We analyze what makes the autistic child happy in order to provoke the desire to progress. A psychologist supervises the work of the users.
ABA is practiced at home, but also in a center. The intervention is at least 15 to 20 hours per week, relayed by the parents at home.
The ABA treatment can vary from 1 year to several years.
There are two main "schools": "classic" ABA which consists of repetition and Verbal Behaviour (VB) where the child first learns to make requests. The autistic child knows how to name an object that is shown to him, but he will not know how to ask for it, so that is the goal of VB.
VB is more widely used than traditional ABA in the United States.
Keep in mind that these are just fads, fashionable trends. The term "ABA" or other doesn't matter,

it's the educator who is the most important, his empathy for your child, his love for him, his willingness, his gift to help the weak and disabled.

If you do not have a good feeling about a professional, it is because he or she is not the right therapist for you, whatever the name of the method used. The human being comes first, not the method.

The problem with ABA is that it invades your life, your space and your time (that of your couple, your relationship with your children, etc.) These therapies, American, correspond well to the need to "appear" in American society. They go to great lengths to make your child appear normal and acceptable. Beware of the overwork and illusions caused by these methods.

honest psychiatrists. They humbly train themselves in other therapies more adapted to autistic people...

Whatever the method...

The most effective programs are based on behavioral approaches.

These programs should focus on :

Improve your relationship with your child

and to

Develop your child's social and communication skills.

The basic principles you should find on these coaching, regardless of the method, are:

1. The adaptation of the method to your child.
2. Regular evaluation of your child's progress.
3. Your participation.

The role of the parents is indeed essential. You need to be helped, supported, and helped to understand your child's behavior and needs.

Exercise 1: Coordinate visual and motor skills.

The child looks at an object.
Reaches for it
And reaches for it.
Child holds the object.
Places it
or takes it out of a box.

Exercise 2: Differentiate one object from another.

The child inserts square objects into square openings,
round objects in round openings,
triangular objects in triangular openings, etc.
This is a first step in learning to sort between different shapes.
The child can then be taught to sort two objects into clear plastic boxes.
For example, your child can learn to put spoons in one box and balls in the other.
Gradually, the child is asked to sort more and more similar objects: spoons and knives rather than spoons and balls.
Then they sort objects of different colors, in opaque boxes, etc.

Exercise 3: Puzzles

Simple puzzles are first of all puzzles with no possible mistakes, where each piece can only fit in one place.

These puzzles can be made easier by copying the visible image on the puzzle piece and placing it in the location where the piece should fit.

Choose puzzles that are compatible with your child's skills; don't challenge him. If he or she is having fun, continue, if not, move on to another game.

Remember, your goal is to make him happy and calm.

Exercise 4: Putting things together

Putting together
objects,
pictures,
identical pictures.

Sorting is an activity that autistic children enjoy because it takes into account their visual skills. Letters and numbers can be sorted. For example, words beginning with "B" and "T" can be sorted into boxes with the letters "B" or "T", etc.

Exercise 5: Eliciting Communication

Put a food that your child really likes in a jar that he or she cannot open.
Show the jar to your child so he or she can see the food. Then put the jar within reach of your child.
See what he does to ask you to give him the food he wants.
Accept all of these gestures as attempts to communicate and give the food to your child.
If your child is not communicating at all, then show him how to communicate by taking his hand and pointing it toward the jar, then give him the food.
By understanding that communication can bring a reward, your child will be more likely to communicate in the future.
Similarly, a toy can be placed in a high place so that your child has to communicate to get it; give the child his favorite puzzle, but keep one piece, so he will have to come to you to get the missing piccc.

Finally, a tickle game can be triggered by a code between you and the child:

"1, 2, 3" or "I'll get you" and then tickle your child if he likes to be tickled.

Repeat until he begins to anticipate that you will tickle him.

Finally, when your child understands the scenario, he will do something to get you to do it again.

Game 4: Imagination Game

Put two different types of toys together in the same activity, such as a character in a car being pushed.
You can also put a doll in a bed and cover it.
The idea is to "pretend".
It is often difficult for children with autism to know how to start an activity.
So you can help your child by posting pictures of available toys on the wall or on the toy box.

Game 5: With other children

When your child has mastered different types of play, you can begin to introduce other children into his or her play.

The other children are gradually integrated:
first in the same room, without interacting ;
then side by side with the same toys, etc.
Sandboxes,
water tables,
Lego boxes,

Theory of Mind: the opposite of autism

Theory of mind is the ability to understand what others think or feel differently than we do.
Theory of mind is used to :
predict the behavior of others
and act accordingly;
explain
and understand one's own behaviors and emotions;
make connections between the behaviors, thoughts and feelings of others.
Theory of mind allows us to perceive the emotions of others,
and understand social rules,
It is used to understand humor, or to identify a lie. It is a basis for social communication.
In text analysis, it would be like answering questions like: "What is the character thinking?", "What would you have done in the place of this character?
The autistic person has, and this is his big problem, difficulty in guessing and understanding what is going on in the minds of others, what they are thinking, feeling, wanting, believing.

So, the theory of mind, you think...

The autistic person's need for immutability

The need for immutability is manifested by a resistance to change,
the systematic recourse to routine activities.
This reassures the autistic person who can thus foresee what will happen. Routine rituals soothe the autistic person.
It is not your child's ill will, a whim, or stubborn behavior.
In order to help the autistic child evolve, a small change can be made from time to time.
We need time and nothing is taken for granted. So if your child has routines and is doing well, let him/her live his/her routine.
After all, we are all routiners, we stay in familiar places and environments.

Perception in detail

Many autistic people focus on details and do not see the big picture.
This prevents them from making sense of situations.
These autistic people are not able to locate the most relevant information.
Well, that's a handicap. But it's not that important. This error of perspective is, in the end, a problem that we encounter everywhere in society. Many of us do not see the overall plan that is being imposed on us.

The "lack of central coherence

The autistic person sees the trees when we see the forest...
Good luck, I have nothing to add!

The importance of visual aids.

Objects, photos, images, pictograms sometimes make information clearer and more accessible for the autistic person and help him/her to be independent.
A picture is worth a thousand words. The autistic person is a "visual thinker".

Visual aids make it possible to retain information and to be able to refer to it at any time. Visual aids have the advantage of being transferable from one context to another.
Visuals can be used anywhere on a schedule, in a binder, on the work table, on the dinner table.

But, frankly, it becomes painful to live with images for parents and siblings... That's it.

What the autistic person expects from us.

The autistic person must be able to anticipate what is expected of him or her and the order in which he or she must perform the activity.
Instructions should use simple vocabulary, even the same words for some, should be affirmative: "Put your pencil on the table" instead of saying "stop playing with your pencil.

What does an autistic person actually expect? It is to be left alone and to live his life.

Recess.

Recess is not a time to relax for an autistic person. The noise, the movements, the absence of reference points, the lack of predictability, make these moments difficult.
The autistic child must be protected from teasing, intimidation, or even abuse by other children during recess, in the bathroom, in the locker room, or during sports class.

It is mandatory for the life assistant to accompany the autistic child at recess, to help with socialization. The autistic child must be allowed a certain amount of freedom, while remaining vigilant. Recess time must be predictable and limited in time. The autistic child must be helped to identify and understand the signals for the beginning and end of playtime.

How to help a hypersensitive autistic child?

For noise, the autistic child can use earplugs or noise-cancelling headphones, or even keep a hood on.
For light, one can use sunglasses, screens.

Sports.

Daily physical activity for more than 20 minutes helps the autistic person reduce stereotyped behaviors, hyperactivity or aggression.
Exercise helps children with autism to better engage with the environment, lose weight and stay healthy like everyone else.
However, sports with other children is more complicated to organize. A space that is too big, noisy, resonant, with too many materials, too much light, reflections, in a new, unstructured place is a source of problems.
The understanding of instructions,
the rules of the sport activity,
waiting,
the collective time (each one in turn),
the difficulty of getting dressed,
to take off one's shoes,
to get dressed, to take off one's shoes, to put on a bathing suit,
getting dressed is a problem...
It is therefore necessary to accompany and supervise.
And, above all, to prepare:
When are we going to do sports?

What are we going to do?
How long will we do it?
Where do we do it?
With whom?
Autistic people often do not belong to a group and do not tolerate losing.
So sports can be considered, but perhaps not a group sport.

How can autism be explained?

Everything can and should be addressed.
We can compare the daily life of a normal person with that of an autistic person.
We can talk about difficulties in relationships with others,
difficulties in communication,
the absence of words, etc.
In any case, you will have two categories around you: intelligent people... And the stupid ones.
I don't waste my time with jerks anymore.

The microbiota.

There is a link between autism and the microbiota, i.e. the microbes contained in the intestines. This concerns the influence of the axis between the intestine and our brain.

A treatment based on Lactobacillus reuteri, an intestinal bacterium contained in yoghurts and maternal milk, could improve social interactions.

Several avenues are being explored. Probiotics, which would improve gastrointestinal disorders and reduce autistic symptoms, is one of them.

Omega-3 supplementation would improve behavior,

a diet free of gluten and milk protein,

as well as a high-fat, low-sugar diet called the "ketogenic diet" would increase sociability and communication skills and decrease stereotyped behaviors.

Fecal microbiota transplantation: no thanks...

This is an experimental therapy in which stool from a healthy donor is introduced into the digestive tract of autistic people in order to rebalance their flora.

This treatment requires the prior intake of antibiotics and a gastric acidity suppressant, a cleaning of the intestines.

The transfer of microbiota is daily for two months.

It's creepy and not really proven to be effective. It's up to you, but...

The role of fluoride.

Prolonged ingestion of fluoride causes significant damage to our health, and in particular to the brain and nervous system.
This could lead to autism.
Tap water and dental products have been fluoridated in Canada and the United States to prevent cavities. This has no effect on tooth decay, but it does damage.
Most countries do not fluoridate their water. Only 11 countries still mandate fluoridated water:
Australia,
Brunei,
Chile,
Guyana,
Hong Kong,
Ireland,
Israel,
Malaysia,
New Zealand,
Singapore
And the United States, of course...
In total, 377,655,000 million people in the world drink artificially fluoridated water, or 5% of the

world's population.

The role of wheat.

Children with autism were found to have significantly higher levels of IgG antibodies to gliadin, the main protein in wheat.
Gluten contains a wide range of peptides (amino acids) that affect neurological, endocrine, immune and digestive health.
Peptides in gluten and casein may play a role in the origins of autism and that the physiology and psychology of autism may be explained by excessive opioid activity related to these peptides. Research has reported abnormal levels of peptides in the urine and cerebrospinal fluid of people with autism.
If this is the case, gluten-free and dairy-free diets should reduce the symptoms associated with autism. A whole-food, natural-fat, grain-free diet is a first step toward improving many ailments, not just in autism.

Probiotics

Probiotics are living microorganisms that may have beneficial effects on the health of the host. The gut and the brain can influence each other. Probiotics can prevent intestinal inflammation or alteration of the microflora and thus preserve the brain.
Two capsules per day of Lactobacillus acidophilus would significantly improve eye contact and correct recognition of human emotion in autistic people.

Equine therapy

Equine therapy has positive effects on autistic people. A peaceful horse or pony is used to ride an autistic person.

The latter learns, in safety, to indulge in the imperatives of horseback riding, to take care of the animal.

Equitherapy is also the most popular animal therapy in autism.

Sugar.

The behavioral effects of high and low blood sugar, cortisol, and insulin account for energy levels, agitation, and hyperactivity.
But there is a more insidious process: sugar causes inflammation and suppresses a growth factor in the brain called BDNF.

Genetically modified foods sprayed with glyphosate

Glyphosate and genetically modified foods wreak havoc on our gut. These chemicals decimate our beneficial bacteria, produce ammonia, interfere with our hormone managing enzymes, etc.
Eliminate these products as much as possible, as well as fermented foods like sauerkraut and pickles from your autistic child's diet.

Industrial food dyes and additives.

Banned in Europe, these food additives impair cognitive function.
Eliminate food coloring,
sodium benzoate,
glutamate and aspartame that cause attention deficits and hyperactivity.

Neurobehavioral abnormalities are attributed to brain-penetrating additives such as:
Polysorbate 80,
aluminum
and mercury.
Hepatitis B vaccination, in particular, is believed to cause hyperactivity and autism.

Melatonin

Many children with autism have problems sleeping. Insomnia can exacerbate many symptoms of autism.
A natural melatonin supplement helps people with autism sleep better.

Chemicals, detergents.

We are poisoned by pesticide residues in our food, pollution in our environment. Autistic people are even more fragile.
It would be advisable to eliminate from our environment the :
Chlorpyrifos,
pesticide called O-diethyl (from Dow Chemical Company...),
Polybrominated diphenyl ethers,
lead,
Methylmercury,
Polychlorinated biphenyls (called "pyralenes" by Monsanto),
Arsenic,
Fluors,
the aromatic hydrocarbon Toluene (called methylbenzene or phenylmethanol.)
Manganese
and the Tetrachloethylene, used for the dry cleaning of fabrics and for degreasing metals.
It would be advisable, above all, that we are informed of all the crap that is put in food products, detergents and all the products of the daily life that the so-called modern society gives

us...

Omega-3.

Autism could be linked to deficiencies in fatty acids rich in omega-3.
A regular cure of these rich essential fatty acids could improve the symptoms.

Chelation

Toxic metals would aggravate autistic symptoms.

Excretion of these heavy metals by using chelating agents to detoxify the body of harmful minerals and metals could lead to an improvement in symptoms.

The chelating agent would bind to electrically charged minerals or metals.

Such as iron,

calcium,

lead,

copper, etc.

This aggregation would give a non-toxic complex which would be eliminated by urinary way.

The chelating agents can be natural (chlorella, coriander). The problem with this method is the elimination. We are not sure that 100% of it is eliminated through the urine without going to other areas of the body.

The ketogenic diet.

A high-fat, moderate-protein, low-carbohydrate, gluten-free, casein-free diet can help people with autism.
The body is forced to use fat instead of glucose for energy.
This means that bread, rice and pasta should not be eaten.
Here are the foods to eat on a ketogenic diet:
nuts and peanuts
eggs
fish (salmon, tuna, sardines, sole, trout)
poultry (chicken, duck, turkey),
meat (beef, veal, lamb, pork)
seafood (shrimp, lobster, crab),
blueberries,
lemon,
olives,
raspberries,
spinach,
broccoli,
beans,
avocado,
lettuce.

Histamine

When we come into contact with an allergen, such as pollen or insect venom, our bodies release histamine to overcome the aggression.
The skin rash, itchy eyes or swelling are produced by histamine.
The autistic person would develop an allergy to histamine.
As a result, their immune system and neurological development are affected.
Sleep disorders,
anxiety,
learning disabilities
and absorption problems are also observed.
Avoid fermented foods:
tea (black/green),
chocolate,
cocoa, cola,
alcoholic beverages. Red wine is particularly high in histamine.

Avoid eating overripe fruits and vegetables, as histamine levels increase as these foods ripen.

Histamine is formed from bacterial action that occurs when food begins to rot.
Drink water to avoid constipation.
Food can begin to ferment in the gut and increase the histamine load in the body.
Favor foods rich in the bioflavonoid luteolin, which help reduce inflammation and curb histamine reactions:
parsley,
artichokes,
celery,
olive oil,
rosemary,
peppermint,
sage
and thyme
are all good sources.
Finally, take 2000 mg of vitamin C daily, as it has natural antihistamine properties.
The brain and gut are particularly susceptible to oxidative damage.
Antioxidants such as vitamin C are effective in reducing the oxidative stress associated with autism.

Computers, tablets.

All parents of autistic children bless tablets and computers, despite their flaws. The professionals who tell us to limit screens in the home do not have children with autism!
We see our children becoming calm, attentive, relaxed in front of their screens. And this allows us to breathe, despite the ayatollahs of our children's education.
It turns out that this has not escaped the attention of researchers.
Children with autism have a special affinity for computers, and current research shows that it is possible to use digital technology to help them develop their social skills.
The advantage of digital technology is that children with autism can experiment with different social scenarios on screens without real risk. They learn without fear of failure.
In the future, computer science could therefore offer autistic people a professional environment favorable to their inclinations. This is an avenue to be explored.

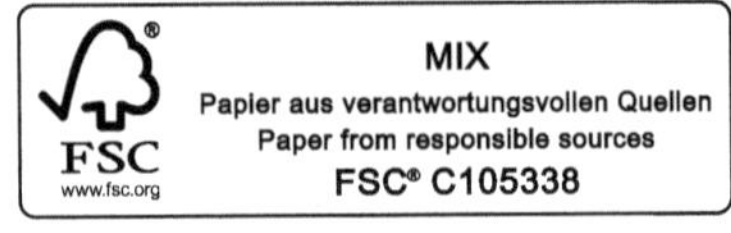

Printed by Books on Demand GmbH, Norderstedt / Germany